C000233572

Th Complete Dr. Sebi Alkaline Diet Guide

Jennifer Thomas

COPYRIGHT PAGE

DEDICATION

I specially dedicate this book to you.

Table of Contents

Contents

INTRODUCTION

Dr. Sebi Approved Detox Guide helps you easy and effective methods for eating with providing comfort and convenience if you have a busy and choked-up lifestyle. Be that as it may, the sort of nourishment available in a hurry will, in general, leave our bodies feeling languid, overloaded and loaded with negative sensations. Inexpensive, fast food, red meat, and greasy/oily nourishments so frequently lead to weight gain, heart issues, medical problems and a reduction in vitality.

What you have before you is the Dr. Sebi's approved Nutritional Guide. It is a complete compilation of all foods and recipes as approved and recommended by Dr. Sebi for all individuals who want to undergo cleansing of their bodies. These foods and recipes are ideal for your alkaline diets in losing weight, staying healthy and revitalizing your body. This list of Dr. Sebi approved foods and recipes will do you some great benefits. Checking them out will improve on your health status.

What are you waiting for? Ready?

Lets' go. Simply click on the download button now.

CHAPTER ONE

DR. SEBI PRODUCTS NUTRITIONAL GUIDE: LIST OF DR SEBI RECOMMENDED FOODS YOU SHOULD TRY TODAY

ALKALINE GRAINS

- Amaranth
- Fonio
- Kamut
- Quinoa
- Rye
- Spelt
- Tef
- Wild Rice

ALL NATURAL HERBAL TEAS

- Burdock
- Chamomile

- Elderberry
- Fennel
- Ginger
- Red Raspberry
- Tila

FRUITS

(No canned fruits or Seedless fruits)

- Apples
- Bananas – the smallest of size
- Berries – all kinds- any form of Elderberries except cranberries
- Cantaloupes
- Cherries
- Currants
- Dates
- Figs
- Grapes – Seeded
- Limes (Key limes preferred with seeds)
- Mangoes
- Melons – Seeded
- Orange (Seville or sour preferred)
- Papayas
- Peaches
- Pears
- Plums

- Prickly Pear (Cactus Fruit)
- Prunes
- Raisins – Seeded
- Soft Jelly Coconuts (and coconut oil)
- Soursops
- Tamarinds

NUTS & SEEDS

(Includes nut & seed butters)

- Brazil Nuts
- Hemp Seeds
- Raw Sesame (Tahini) Butter
- Raw Sesame Seeds
- Walnuts

OILS

Minimize the use of oils.

- Avocado Oil
- Coconut Oil (Do not cook)
- Grapeseed Oil
- Hempseed Oil
- Olive Oil (Do not cook)
- Sesame Oil

SPICES – SEASONINGS

- Achiote
- Basil
- Bay leaf
- Cayenne/African Bird Pepper
- Cloves
- Dill
- Habanero
- Onion Powder
- Oregano
- Powdered Granulated Seaweed (Kelp/Dulce/Nori)
- Pure Sea Salt
- Sage
- Savory
- Sweet Basil
- Tarragon
- Thyme

SUGARS

- 100% Pure Agave Syrup
- Date sugar – (sources should be dried dates)

VEGETABLES

- Amaranth greens (Callaloo)
- Avocado
- Bell Peppers
- Chayote (Mexican Squash)
- Cucumber
- Dandelion greens
- Garbanzo beans (Chickpeas)
- Izote (Cactus flower/ Cactus leaf)
- Kale
- Lettuce (all, except Iceberg)
- Mushrooms (all, except Shitake)
- Nopal (Mexican Cactus)
- Okra
- Olives (and olive oil)
- Onions
- Purslane (Verdolaga)
- Sea Vegetables (Seamoss/Wakame/Dulse/Arame/Hijiki/Nori)
- Squash
- Tomatillo
- Tomato (Cherry and plum only)
- Turnip greens
- Watercress
- Zucchini

CHAPTER TWO

AN SNEAK REVIEW OF 10 POWERFUL CANCER-KILLING ALKALINE FOODS

Berries and Red wines are great source of anti-oxidants as we all know. Free radicals that causes cancer in the body system are best fought with these anti-oxidants. But individuals are not aware or probably having little awareness about cancer-combating diets enhance battling against cancer and also making you stay healthy.

The speed at which cancer spreads is shown by many scientist/medical researches. It is confirmed and proven that 1:2 (i.e.one out of two men) is likely to develop cancer throughout their lifespan and for the women; the ratio is confirmed that 1:3(i.e. one out of every three women) are also prone to developing cancer. Cancer affects man directly or indirectly and it is a very serious disease. Over 9,000 cancer cells are developed by the average people. These cancer cells must be battled by the body's immune system.

But there is a bigger danger when the body's immune system is unable to combat these cancer cells.

Cancer is a disease that grows gradually over time and certainly it grows completely and it is very dangerous because it is not a disease that one can wake up to find out. What a terrific danger? A bigger hazard is that current advanced technologies at times do not notice this cancer cells in the body until they grow and mature till after eight years.

Therefore the book you want to read now will be perhaps one of the best you will read this year. That is why in this book I will let you know the effective top 10 alkaline foods which will help you fight cancer cells in your body system and also why each of the alkaline foods is very important and necessary for you to include in your daily diet. Let's do this!

1. Beans

2. Broccoli

3. Curcumin

4. Dark, leafy greens

5. Detox tea

6. Garlic

7. Ginger

8.   Healthy Fats

9.   Pistachios, Macadamia Nuts, and Almonds

10   Tomatoes

CHAPTER THREE

THE TRUTHS ABOUT THE TOP 10 ALKALINE DIETS GOOD FOR CANCER CURE

1. BEANS

Beans is a good way to combat cancer. They combat cancer in over one way, one is that they multiply the body system's level of fatty acid which will eventually reduce the growth of cancer in the body.

Another way is that they aid the body in executing toxic substances from the body and taking in nutrients into the body system.

Beans are very good and confirmed to combat colon and breast cancer. It is advisable to add beans to your alkaline diet daily intake cause bean are Alkaline.

2. BROCCOLI

The Broccoli is a marvelous food. It contain more of sulforaphane than other vegetables of it class. It destroys cancer-causing cells by going after them once taken. It also aims terminates developing cells.

If you want to eat more of Broccoli, add it to quinoa bowl, by so doing, you will stir, fry raw soup recipes so that you can get enough out of it.

3. CURCUMIN

The Curcumin is an essential constituent in the spice turmeric. It is very important place in preventing cancer in the body. It makes it virtually impossible and extremely hard for cancer cells to grow, mature or develop in the body because it hugely decreases swellings in the body.

Curcumin deals successfully in combating against bladder and gastrointestinal cancer cells. Curcumin is one of the most effectual cancer-fighting food you need to include in your alkaline diet now.

You can add a pinch black pepper in order to make curcumin active in fighting against cancer.

4. DARK, LEAFY GREENS

Examples of dark, leafy greens that you should have to help you combat cancer cells in alkaline diet includes:

(i) Collard greens

(ii) Kale

(iii) Romaine Lettuce

(iv) Spinach

(v) Swiss Chard

(vi) Turnip

(vii) Watercress

(viii) Any other dark leafy green that you know.

One characteristics about these dark, leafy greens that make them perfect in combating cancer in the body is that they have sufficient and excess folic acid in them which is known as 'Foliate'. Folic acid has the B-

Vitamin which cannot make cells transform into cancer cells. Foliate is very useful in fighting colorectal and pancreatic cells. It is therefore important that you eat dark, leafy greens to fight cancer in your body. And also, you can add these dark, leafy greens to your salad and then your juice and smoothie.

5. DETOX TEA

Researches have revealed that drinking tea decreases the rate of been infected with cancer. You must take tea daily most especially in the morning.

Flavonoids are present in tea. Flavonoids contains anti-oxidants that shields the body from cancer. Medical researches revealed taking tea helps a lot to reduce the danger of breast and ovarian cancer.

Taking of Detox tea every day is advised. You can also add it into your alkaline diet. Hot and Cold teas contain flavonoids so it will be good if you take tea daily throughout the year. Cancer cells will be eliminated from your body within a short period of time.

6. GARLIC

Garlic is a very lovely food. If you like eating garlic, I have a great information for you. It aids in combatting cancer effectively.

Gastrointestinal cancers like intestine, colon, stomach and oesophagal cancer chances, are reduced whenever you take in 'Garlic' in your body.

You can also add garlic to dips like salad, hummus, and guacamole and tomato sauce.

7. GINGER

Another effectual eliminator of cancerous cells is Ginger. It is also a best substitute to cure cancer patients when chemotherapy seems not to be effective.

It has the power to eliminate definite types of cancer cells like the ovarian cancer. So the ginger is essential in fighting cancer in the body system and not just a spice for comfort.

What you need to do is to eat ginger
by putting it in your soup, smoothies
and your dishes. It is also useful as a
sweetener in desserts. It is advised
that you take in more of ginger.

It is preferably that you take your
canned tomatoes every day in your
alkaline diet and also you you add it
in your pasta dishes and your raw and
hot soups.

8. HEALTHY FATS

Most people avoid fats when it comes
to avoiding and eliminating cancer.
The true fact is that healthy fats aids
fighting cancer.

Extra virgin olive oil and coconut oil are potent healthy oils that effective in combating cancer. They are effectual cancer avoiders which keep the human body healthy.

Therefore, it is advised that you take in more of these fats. You can do this by adding seeds and coconut oil to smoothie you eat every day.

9. PISTACHIOS, MACADAMIA NUTS, AND ALMONDS

These nuts are extremely rich phytosterols. They are very suitable in combating cancer cells. Their job is to prevent estrogen receptors that are present in breast cancers. are good at wrestling against cancer cells.

It is an absolute prospect that the rate of prostate cancer amidst people and stopping cancer growth with these nuts. You can also eat these nuts by adding it to your granola and smoothies' salads.

10. TOMATOES

Tomatoes have stupendous health advantages. Through medical researchers, they are very useful in killing cancer cells. They also aid avoiding the developing of cancer in the Prostate gland, stomach and in the lungs.

It is suggested that you take more tomato daily and you can also add it to your alkaline diet. Lycopene has been confirmed to be available in canned tomatoes.

CHAPTER FOUR

DR. SEBI HERBS: 4 POWERFUL APPROVED FOR YOUR ALKALINE DIET

There are two proportions to healing the body:

1. Cleanse the body

2. Revitalize the body

Dr. Sebi has suggested 4 strong plants that can help you succeed in accomplishing the renewing of your emerging and also cleansing your body system.

Dr. Sebi herbs: 4 Powerful Herbs recommended by Dr. Sebi

These herbs, as approved by Dr. Sebi are effective. They are commonly found in the African continent, specifically in the African forests. In such habitats, you will discover four beneficial plants. which are:

1.   Cancansa

2.   Hoodia

3.   Iboga

4.   She-Saw

1. The Cancansa

The Cancansa herb is a strong and powerful plant for the grown-up. It is very advantageous for adults who are 90 years old and above. At these ages, you will see that you are shortfall, particularly in the aspect of sexuality. There is no cause for anxiety, just take this herb to gain renewal in your sexual vigor. You get immediate sexual energy once you take it. Absolute, you just read that– instantaneous sexual energy renewal, that is how influential it is.

2. The Hoodia Herb

Namibia a country in Africa is a popular place to find another potent herb called Hoodia. The plant give sufficient nutrients to the body. When you take it, you don't have to eat for days because it is capable of nourishing the body.

3. The Iboga Herb

The herb Iboga is found in Cameroon and it is the most powerful and influential herb which helps in the calming of the human system which gives the body a state of atmospheric enjoyment. The powerful herb is useful for those with emotive problems.

4. The She-Haw Herb

The She-Haw herb is seen in the wilds of Africa which is also an influential herb. It offers substantial profits to many people across the world, Michael Jackson's son . It has provides significant benefits to many individuals across the world. The world-famous Michael Jackson's son profited from it because he was chanced to use it when he had a tumor in the frontal lobe of his body. He sneezed the tumor out not less than 20 minutes that he took it. You can now see how potent the herb is.

CHAPTER FIVE

7 BEST DR. SEBI APPROVED ALKALINE RECIPES

RECIPE 1: Cellular Level Mixed Berry Smoothie

Ingredients

(i) 1 tablespoon raw agave

(ii) 1-2 teaspoons of sea moss powder or sea moss gel

(iii) 1/8 cup of fresh blueberries

(iv) ¼ cup sliced yellow banana (burro)

(v) 1 tablespoon of raw hemp seeds

(vi) ½ cup of sliced fresh strawberries

(vii) ½ cup fresh raspberries

Directions

(i) Keep some berries aside to be used after you get your finished smoothie.

(ii) Combine banana, the remnant raspberries and strawberries. Blend them together until they are smooth.

(iii)   Pour the gotten smoothie into a bowl.

(iv)   Carefully arrange the earlier kept blueberries, berries and hemp seeds on top of the smoothie.

(v) Use the agave to drizzle.

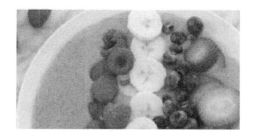

RECIPE 2: Mango Sherbet

Ingredients

(i) 2 mangoes

(ii) ½ cup of coconut milk

(iii)   ¼ cup of agave

Directions

(i) Cut the two mangoes into small pieces.

(ii) Freeze them up for about 8 hours.

(iii)   After 8 hours of freezing, blend them.

(iv)   Add the coconut milk

(v) Add the ¼ cup of agave.

(vi)   Stir and serve.

(vii)   Enjoy with your loved ones.

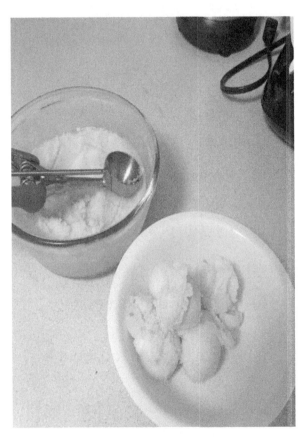

RECIPE 3: Hemp Milk Recipe

Ingredients

(i) Pinch of sea salt

(ii) ½ cup of hemp seeds

(iii)   2 tablespoons of date syrup

(iv)   3 to 4 cups of water

Directions

(i) Gather all the above ingredients together.

(ii) Blend them in a good blender with high speed.

(iii)   Strain off water.

(iv)   Store in a glass jar and get it refrigerated for 5 days.

(v) Serve chilled and enjoy.

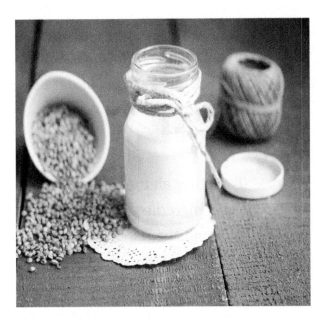

Ingredients

(i) 1 cup of mushrooms

(ii) ¼ cup of Quinoa

(iii)   1 cup of soaked Garbanzo beans

(iv)   ¼ cup of onions

(v) ¼ cup of Garbanzo bean flour

(vi)   ¼ cup of pepper

(vii)   Your favorite alkaline
        seasoning

Directions

(i) Combine all the above
        ingredients together.
(ii) Blend them in a blender or
        food processor.
(iii)   Mold to your desired size.
(iv)   Fry in a frying pan
(v) Alternatively, you can bake in a
        pre-heated hot oven.

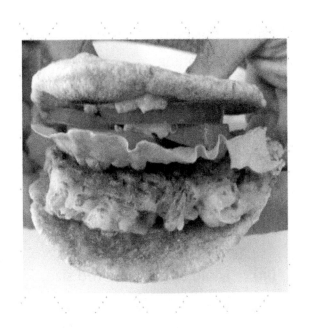

RECIPE 5: Alkaline Hot Sauce

Ingredients

(i) 1 ½ cups of spring water

(ii) ½ cup of hey lime juice

(iii) 9 plum tomatoes

(iv) 1 ½ teaspoon of sea salt

(v) 1 tablespoon of sea moss
powder

(vi)   2 tablespoons of onion powder

(vii)   2 tablespoons of cayenne pepper

Directions

(i) Combine all ingredients together.

(ii) Blend them in a blender.

(iii)   Cook on a medium heated oven for 15 minutes.

(iv)   You can decide to add more water to make it less thick.

(v) Take a little over 1 cup.

(vi)   Serve and enjoy.

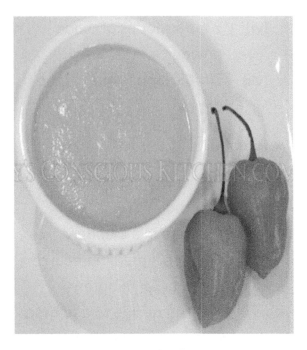

RECIPE 6: Alkaline Chickpea Fritters

Ingredients

   (i) ½ cup of garbanzo bean flour

   (ii) ½ teaspoon of spring water

   (iii)   Or 1/8 cup of spring water

Directions

(i) Add your preferred alkaline seasoning and veggies in combination with the above ingredients.

(ii) Thoroughly mix ingredients together and fry in an alkaline oil (i.e. Sesame or grape seed)

(iii)   Serve and enjoy.

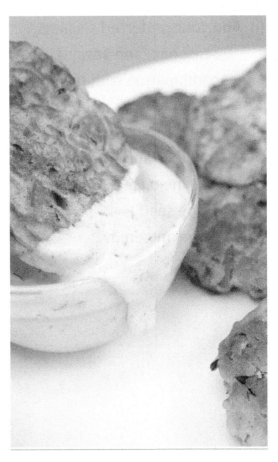

RECIPE 7: Alkaline Corn Bread

Ingredients

   (i) 2 cups of chickpea flour.

(ii) 1 cup of applesauce (you can easily get an applesauce by blending 2 apples to make a puree).

(iii)   ½ Cup of G.S. oil

(iv)   1 tablespoon of green pepper

(v) 1 cup of Brazilnut milk

(vi)   Water as needed.

Directions

(i) Mix all ingredients together.

(ii) Use spring water to thin out.

(iii)   Oil pan with grape seed oil and add batter.

(iv)   Bake on 325 degree pre-heated oven for 30 minutes.

(v) Serve and enjoy.

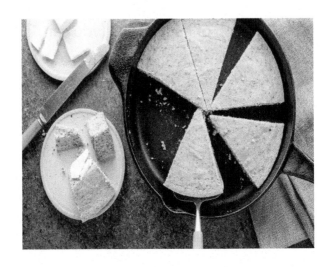

BONUS CHAPTER

5 ESSENTIAL OILS FOR WEIGHT LOSS

We all know that oil taken from plant is free from any bad condition from felling any sickness or headache. There are something to show you that the oil is good when you smell, when you it to cook food or you put on any surface of iron, it also assist to reduce cholesterol and fat. Add to weight and energy. If you have good health and you always do exercise many of the oil we assist you in burning of your fat.

ESSENTIAL OIL 1: LEMON OIL

Lemon oil is good oil that helps in weight loss, lemon good oil assist detoxification, and it helps to build up inside body and it will reduce the power of poisonous food.

Removing all the poisonous substances in your body will make you look so young. It will reduce fat and increase the energy in your body. In addition, it assists the white blood cells from wasting. It will free your body from sickness and other health problem.

ESSENTAIL OIL 2: LAVENDER OIL

When reaching out for your favorite food when you are over stressed, use lavender oil. It helps in relaxation and reduces tension in the body and it helps to give restful sleep.

It helps to reduce an unhealthy skin, so we need oil like lavender oil to satisfy our wants. Using the oil will help us in relaxing.

ESSENTAIL OIL 3: GRAPEFRUIT OIL

Grapefruit oil is very good for the body. Much thanks to all the scientific talks about it. The oil burns body fat.

Grapefruit and grapefruit oil helps in breaking down the body fat in quick action. It allows the tissue to receive nutrient thereby giving power to the body to save you from all sickness that can enter the body. It also reduces the fat of the stomach.

Not all oils are safe for the skin but the grapefruit oil has proven to be excellent for the human body. It will surely do you good. You can use grapefruit to reduce hunger by putting one drop to a cup of water.

ESSENTAIL OIL 4: HOLY BASIL OIL

Holy basil oil helps in reducing stress when you pass through too much stress. It reduces emotional stress and worries.

It can also add to weight-loss. It helps in brain activity. When picking the best oils for weight loss, the Holy Basil oil will surely take its rightful place.

ESSENTAIL OIL 5: GINGER OIL

Ginger oil is very good for digestion and reduction of injuries in the body. It also helps reduce sugar in the body. It helps to reduce fat in the body and the ability of your brain.

Adding two drops to the water you want to use to bath and putting it to the tea you want to drink or taking the smell directly from the bottle will do much good to you. It is good very for the health.

OTHER BOOKS BY THE AUTHOR

Printed in Great Britain
by Amazon

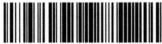

35956357R00037